Paleo Diet Cookbook

50+ Healthy Paleo-Friendly Recipes for Breakfast, Lunch, Dinner, and Dessert

© **Copyright 2017 by John Carter - All rights reserved.**

This document is geared towards providing exact and reliable information in regards to the topic and issue covered. The publication is sold with the idea that the publisher is not required to render accounting, officially permitted, or otherwise, qualified services. If advice is necessary, legal or professional, a practiced individual in the profession should be ordered.

- From a Declaration of Principles which was accepted and approved equally by a Committee of the American Bar Association and a Committee of Publishers and Associations.

In no way is it legal to reproduce, duplicate, or transmit any part of this document in either electronic means or in printed format. Recording of this publication is strictly prohibited and any storage of this document is not allowed unless with written permission from the publisher. All rights reserved.

The information provided herein is stated to be truthful and consistent, in that any liability, in terms of inattention or otherwise, by any usage or abuse of any policies, processes, or directions contained within is the solitary and utter responsibility of the recipient reader. Under no circumstances will any legal responsibility or blame be held against the publisher for any reparation, damages, or monetary loss due to the information herein, either directly or indirectly.

Respective authors own all copyrights not held by the publisher.

The information herein is offered for informational purposes solely, and is universal as so. The presentation of the information is without contract or any type of guarantee assurance.

The trademarks that are used are without any consent, and the publication of the trademark is without permission or backing by the trademark owner. All trademarks and brands within this book are for clarifying purposes only and are the owned by the owners themselves, not affiliated with this document.

Bonus:
FREE Report Reveals
The Secrets To Lose Weight

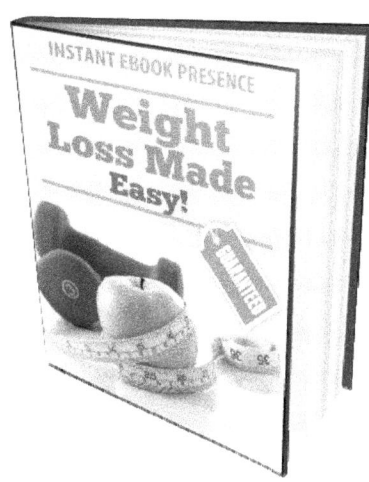

Weight loss doesn't happen from dieting only. Diets are short term solutions to shed extra weight. Diets do not work in the long term because people hate being on a diet (it's ok, you can admit that here). The only long term solution for permanent weight loss is to create new eating habits. This doesn't mean that chocolate will never pass your lips again, but it does mean looking after yourself and watching what you eat...

You can lose weight when you have the right reasons and motivation, and a part of this guide is to help you to find the motivation you need to change your weight...

Get This Guide For FREE
www.sportsforsoul.com/weight-loss-2/

Table Of Contents

Introduction 1

Chapter 1: A Brief Overview of Everything You Need to Know About the Paleo Diet 2

Benefits of the Paleo Diet 3

#1: The Paleo Diet is For Anyone 3

#2: The Paleo Diet is Satiating 3

#3: The Paleo Diet Can Manage and Prevent Some Diseases 3

#5: The Paleo Diet Improves Your Energy 4

Basic Guidelines for the Paleo Diet 4

Chapter 2: Paleo Breakfast Recipes 6

Apple Cinnamon 'Faux'tmeal 6

Vegetarian Leek Frittata Topped with Arugula Salad 7

Coconut Chia Berry Smoothie 9

Banana Carrot Muffins 10

Vegan Zucchini and Pumpkin Muffins 11

Avocado Shrimp Omelet 13

Savory Sausage-Zucchini Casserole 15

Deconstructed BLT Topped with Eggs 17

Chorizo Scramble 18

Coconut-Cinnamon Pancakes 19

Almond Butter and Apple Smoothie 20

Paleo Burger with Eggs and Cashew Cheese 21

Chapter 3: Paleo Main Course Recipes 23

Smoked Salmon with Dill and Fennel 23

Garlic-Ginger Pork Tenders over Cauliflower Rice 24

Paleo Portobello BLT 26

Danish Meatloaf 27

Sweet and Savory Cacao Nip Pork Chops with Butternut Squash 29

Springtime Pasta with Shrimp and Asparagus 31

Beef and Vegetable Asian-Style Wrap 33

Coconut and Lemongrass Chicken Drumsticks...................................... 35

Hearty Turkey Chili.. 37

Creamy Broccoli and Chicken Casserole 39

Crock Pot Kalua Pig 41

Roasted Tomatoes Stuffed with Sausage 42

Crunchy Chicken Fingers... 43

Sage-Infused Portobello and Beef Burgers 45

Rosemary Grilled Chicken Breast Wrapped with Bacon........................ 46

Creamy Coconut Clam Chowder 47

Beef and Liver Mediterranean-Style Eggplant.. 49

Cilantro Lime Pork Tacos 51

Paleo Supreme Pizza.. 53

Chapter 4: Paleo Sides, Soups, Dips, Dressings, and Salads 55

Zucchini Fritters... 55

Avocado-Cilantro Dressing/Dip.. 57

Sautéed Sweet Potatoes... 58

Basic Salad Dressing 59

Apple Coleslaw 60

Creamy Garlic-Pepper Dip.. 61

Shrimp Cakes 62

Paleo Langostino Lobster Squat Soup 63

Creamy Mushroom Soup 65

Garlic-Ginger Almond Dressing.. 66

Sweet Potato Fries 67

Roasted Roots Ratatouille 68

Italian-Style Garlic and Herb Spaghetti Squash 69

Simple Cauliflower Rice 70

Paleo Mayonnaise 71

Paleo Egg Drop Soup 72

French Dressing 73

Paleo Bread 74

Broccoli Soup 75

Chapter 5: Paleo Snacks and Desserts 77

Bacon Wrapped Dates 77

Coconut Cashew Cream and Banana Tart 78

Guacamole Deviled Eggs 80

Spiced Pumpkin Seeds 81

Dehydrated Apple Chips 83

Chocolate-Coconut No-Bakes 84

Cucumber Salmon Bites with Cashew Cheese 85

Easy Watermelon Freeze 87

Sweet Potato Brownies and Chocolate Icing 88

Paleo Trail Mix 90

'Ice Cream' Bites 91

Bacon-Tomato Sweet Potato Bites 92

Strawberry Rhubarb Crisp 93

Coconut Whipped Cream 95

Almond Macaroons 96

Chia Seed Pudding with Coconut and Pecans 97

Conclusion 99

Introduction

I want to thank you and congratulate you for downloading the book, *"Paleo Diet: A Guide to the Paleo Diet with 50+ Recipes for Breakfast, Lunch, Dinner, and Dessert"*.

This book contains proven steps and strategies on how to eat on the Paleolithic Diet. The Paleo Diet is about resetting the body so it functions at its highest level of health. Eating a diet similar to the one eaten by our caveman ancestors, hundreds of centuries ago, does this. It includes foods that can be found in nature, like fruits and vegetables, nuts, and meats.

The Paleo Diet has many benefits, including improving weight loss efforts, fighting inflammation throughout the body, boosting energy, and more. You will learn more about the benefits and guidelines of the Paleo Diet in the first chapter.

The best part is you do not have to suffer- you can even enjoy desserts when they are made with wholesome ingredients. You will find recipes for these scrumptious desserts, as well as for every other meal of the day in the pages of this book.

Thanks again for downloading this book, I hope you enjoy it!

Chapter 1: A Brief Overview of Everything You Need to Know About the Paleo Diet

Before the agricultural revolution, about 10,000 years ago, people ate what is now called the Paleolithic Diet. This diet is also often referred to as the hunter-gatherer diet or the caveman diet since it is made up mostly of meats, fruits and vegetables, and nuts. The Paleo Diet is one free of refined products like artificial sugars and refined grains. It focuses on eating wholesome, nutrient rich foods to fill you up without filling up your waistline.

The Paleo Diet was introduced in the 1970s, though only the recent decade has shown a widespread interest in the diet. The major idea is that the human body can return to a better state of health by returning to eating at its roots- during the caveman era. This chapter will teach you what you need to know about the Paleo Diet, including its health benefits and some basic guidelines before jumping into the recipe portion of the book.

Benefits of the Paleo Diet

Some of the benefits of the Paleo Diet include:

#1: The Paleo Diet is For Anyone
The Paleo Diet fits a wide range of health needs. Since it focuses on eating wholesome foods, rather than eating a certain calorie range, the diet can be adjusted to suit the needs of someone looking to lose weight, athletes, or even the average person who just wants to be healthier.

#2: The Paleo Diet is Satiating
Unlike many diets, you do not have to go hungry when you eat Paleo. The foods that you eat are high in nutrients, protein, and healthy fats. This means that you (and your body) are more satisfied and you are more likely to eat less.

#3: The Paleo Diet Can Manage and Prevent Some Diseases
The Paleo Diet has been deeply studied in the past few decades, most of the research showing promising results for many things. Eating a diet low in processed and refined foods has shown reduced risk of heart disease, improved cholesterol levels, and management of Type 2 diabetes.

#4: The Paleo Diet Has Anti-Inflammatory Benefits
The Paleo Diet is built on the principle that people's diets have evolved more than their bodies. Part of this is a sensitivity to things like gluten and dairy. Since the Paleo Diet removes these foods, it has an anti-inflammatory benefit on the body. People following this diet also frequently eat fruits and vegetables that contain antioxidants, which fight inflammation throughout the body.

#5: The Paleo Diet Improves Your Energy

When you eat better, your body will feel better. Since the foods you eat on the Paleo Diet are full of nutrients, vitamins, and minerals, your body has better sources to burn as full. This can stop fatigue and help power you through a workout. Additionally, you will sleep better since your energy levels are stabilized throughout the day.

Basic Guidelines for the Paleo Diet

Following the Paleo Diet is rather simple- just avoid refined grains, sugars, processed foods, and other foods that were not around when your ancestors lived 10,000 years ago. Most people on the Paleo Diet also avoid dairy products, especially those that are highly processed.

In addition to avoiding processed foods, you should choose meats, fruits, and vegetables from organic sources. Organically-sourced foods are important. You should also try to purchase grass-fed beef and other foods, rather than grain-fed since grain-fed animals have many of the same problems as grain-fed humans.

Foods to Eat

The foods that you should eat on the Paleo Diet include:

- Lean meats
- Nuts and seeds
- Fruits and vegetables
- Seafood
- Healthy fats

Foods to Avoid

The foods to avoid on the Paleo Diet include:

- Grains (especially refined grains)
- Sugars
- Processed foods
- Starches
- Legumes
- Dairy
- Alcohol
- Coffee

You may be looking over the list above and wondering how you can possibly make a meal out of those types of foods. The following chapters in this book will provide you with delicious recipes, for every meal of the day and even dessert that include healthy, Paleo-friendly ingredients. Enjoy!

Chapter 2: Paleo Breakfast Recipes

Apple Cinnamon 'Faux'tmeal

This sweet and spicy 'oatmeal' will satisfy your warm, breakfast cereal craving. You can top with your choice of extra apples, cinnamon, raisins, or nuts.

Ingredients (for 1 serving)

- 1 ½ cups unsweetened applesauce
- ½ cup chunky almond butter
- ¼ cup full-fat coconut milk
- 1 ½ teaspoons cinnamon (or to taste)
- ½ teaspoon ground nutmeg

Instructions

Add all the ingredients to a small pan and warm over medium heat. Stir frequently as you cook for about 10 minutes, until all the ingredients are warm and thoroughly combined. Stir in your choice of toppings before serving.

Vegetarian Leek Frittata Topped with Arugula Salad

This vegetarian Paleo recipe has plenty of flavors. It is great for weekends, but also quick enough that you can put together for a week morning.

Ingredients (for 8 servings)

For the frittata:

- 12 eggs
- ½ cup full-fat coconut milk
- ¼ cup coconut oil
- 1 small leek (sliced)
- 2 cloves garlic (minced)
- ¼ teaspoon salt
- 1/8 teaspoon pepper

For the arugula salad:

- 4 cups baby arugula (loosely packed)
- ½ cup grape tomatoes (halved)
- 1 1/2 tablespoons olive oil
- 3/4 teaspoon balsamic vinegar

Instructions

Set the oven to 350 to preheat. Then, add the coconut milk to a medium bowl and add the salt. Mix this together before whisking the eggs in, beating until well combined.

Add the coconut oil to a cast iron skillet over medium heat. Cook about 5 minutes, until softened. Then, add the garlic and cook until fragrant, about 1 minute longer. Pour the eggs into the skillet and add the pepper and additional salt, to taste. Cook for 20-25 minutes, until just set. Do not overcook the frittata or it will become rubbery.

When the frittata is almost done, whisk together the balsamic vinegar and olive oil. Allow the frittata to sit for 5 minutes once it comes out of the oven and then top with the arugula, halved tomatoes, and dressing.

Coconut Chia Berry Smoothie

Ripe, flavorful berries of your choice come together with assorted fruits and veggies, as well as coconut milk for healthy fats and chia seeds for an extra boost of protein. It's a great way to start the morning.

Ingredients (for 2 servings)

- 1 cup frozen berries of your choice
- 2 cups baby spinach leaves
- 1 banana
- ¼ cup full-fat coconut milk
- 3 tablespoons chia seeds
- 1 teaspoon coconut oil

Instructions

Chop the banana into pieces and add it with all the other ingredients to a blender. Process until the smoothie reaches your desired consistency, adding water as necessary to help with the blending process. You can top with additional chia seeds, coconut flakes, and berries if you would like.

Banana Carrot Muffins

Unlike most flour-free muffins, these are incredibly moist. They are also packed full of nutrients, healthy fats, and protein.

Ingredients (for 12 servings)

- 2 cups almond flour
- 1 ½ cups shredded carrots
- 3 eggs
- 3 bananas
- 1 cup dates (pitted)
- ¾ cup walnuts
- ¼ cup coconut oil (melted)
- 2 tablespoons baking soda
- 1 tablespoon cinnamon
- 1 teaspoon apple cider vinegar
- 1 teaspoon salt

Instructions

Set the oven to 350 degrees to preheat. Sift the flour, cinnamon, baking soda, and salt into a large bowl and set to the side. Then, add the dates, eggs, bananas, coconut oil, and vinegar to a food processor and pulse until blended and well combined.

Add the banana-date mixture to the flour bowl you set aside. Mix to combine thoroughly. Then, fold the carrots and walnuts into the mixture, being sure not to over combine. Use a spoon to fill 12 paper-lined muffin tins. Bake the muffins for 25 minutes, until firmed all the way through.

Vegan Zucchini and Pumpkin Muffins

This is another moist, delicious muffin recipe. This one is free of eggs and milk, making it completely vegan. It is especially tasty in the fall, giving you a low-carb way to enjoy pumpkin spice flavors.

Ingredients (for 6 servings)

- 1 cup almond flour
- ½ cup tapioca flour
- ½ cup coconut flour
- 2 cups pumpkin puree
- 1 cup dates (pitted)
- ½ cup frozen mixed berries
- 1 small zucchini (grated)
- ¾ cup almonds (sliced)
- ¼ cup coconut oil
- 6 tablespoons water
- 2 tablespoons flax seeds (ground)
- 1 tablespoon allspice
- 1 tablespoon cinnamon
- 2 teaspoons baking soda
- 1 teaspoon apple cider vinegar
- 1 teaspoon salt

Instructions

Set the oven to 350 degrees to preheat. Add the water and flax meal to a small bowl and let sit for about 5 minutes, until they have a gooey consistency. While you are waiting, sift the three flours, allspice, cinnamon, baking soda, and salt to a large bowl and mix to combine. Set this to the side.

Take a food processor and pulse the pumpkin, dates, flax meal mixture, coconut oil, and apple cider vinegar until the dates are roughly chopped. Fold this into the dry mixture, being sure not to over-stir.

Then, fold in the zucchini, berries, and nuts. Place the finished mixture into 6 paper-lined muffin tins and bake for 25 minutes, until firm all the way through.

Avocado Shrimp Omelet

Shrimp isn't a common omelet ingredient, but this recipe will have you wondering why you've never tried it. It's a great way to start the day, plus the avocado and shrimp provide all the right kinds of fat.

Ingredients (for 2 servings)

- 4 eggs (beaten)
- ¼ pound shrimp (de-veined, peeled, tails off)
- ½ avocado (pitted, peeled, and diced)
- 1 tomato (diced)
- 1 tablespoon fresh cilantro (chopped)
- 1 teaspoon coconut oil
- ½ teaspoon salt
- ¼ teaspoon pepper

Instructions

Warm a large skillet over medium heat, greasing if necessary, and cook the shrimp until pink all the way through. Chop and set to the side while you prepare the rest of the omelet.

Then, add half the salt to the beaten eggs and set to the side. Warm a skillet over medium high heat and add the coconut oil once it reaches temperature. Then, pour the eggs inside, tilting the pan around so the egg evenly coats the bottom of the pan.

While you are waiting for the egg to cook, toss the diced tomatoes and avocadoes with the cilantro. Add salt and pepper to taste and set to the side. When the omelet has firmed almost all the way through, add the shrimp to half the omelet. Fold it in half and cook an additional 1-2 minutes. Then, carefully remove from the pan and top with the avocado-tomato mixture you set aside.

Savory Sausage-Zucchini Casserole

This breakfast casserole features flavorful sausage and tender zucchini, all held together with eggs. Some of its other savory flavors come from mushrooms and thyme.

Ingredients (for 4 servings)

- 1 pound breakfast sausage (ground)
- 3 medium zucchini
- 6 cremini mushrooms (halved)
- 1 onion (quartered)
- 6 eggs
- 2 tablespoons almond flour
- 2 teaspoons fresh thyme (chopped)
- ½ teaspoon garlic
- ¼ teaspoon cayenne pepper
- ¼ teaspoon salt

Instructions

Set the oven to 400 degrees to preheat. Then, put the zucchini, mushrooms, and onions into a food processor with a grater blade (you could also grate the veggies by hand). Once the vegetables are grated, use a paper towel to remove excess moisture. Add this to a greased 8x8 baking dish by spreading it evenly across the bottom.

Then, crumble the raw breakfast sausage on top of the vegetables. Sprinkle the top with the almond flour and then the thyme. Set this to the side while you combine the eggs with the garlic, cayenne, and salt in a bowl. Whisk about 30 seconds, until the eggs are a uniform color. Pour this over the vegetables and sausage.

Place the pan in the oven and cook for about 50 minutes, until the top is browned and the sausage and eggs are cooked through. If you notice water, do not worry- this is from the vegetables dehydrating as they cook. Allow the casserole to cool at least 15 minutes before serving.

Deconstructed BLT Topped with Eggs

Who doesn't love crispy bacon, crisp lettuce, and juicy tomatoes? This spin-on-a-classic skips on the grain products and adds avocadoes, crunchy almonds, and bacon grease-fried eggs to the mix.

Ingredients (for 2 servings)

- 6 slices raw bacon (diced)
- 4 eggs
- 1 avocado (peeled, pitted, and sliced)
- 1 cup cherry tomatoes (halved)
- 2 cups baby spinach
- 1 ½ tablespoons almonds (sliced)

Instructions

Add the bacon to a skillet that has been warmed to medium-low heat. Cook for about 15 minutes, stirring often. Take 1 tablespoon of the grease and set it aside for later.

Add the tomatoes and spinach to the pan with the bacon and toss 2-3 minutes, until the tomatoes are warm and the spinach has wilted. While you are waiting for the spinach and tomatoes to cook, warm a second pan over medium heat and fry the eggs, using the reserved bacon grease.

Distribute the bacon, spinach, and tomato mixture onto 4 plates. Top with the eggs, followed by the avocado and almonds.

Chorizo Scramble

This dish features spicy chorizo and fluffy eggs with accents of red peppers and onions. Top with fresh salsa and/or cilantro for serving.

Ingredients (for 2 servings)

- 4 eggs
- ½ pound chorizo (no filler ingredients, sliced)
- 1 red bell pepper (diced)
- ½ onion (diced)
- 1 tablespoon coconut oil
- ¼ teaspoon salt
- ¼ teaspoon pepper
- ¼ teaspoon hot sauce (or to taste)

Instructions

Place a saute pan on the stove and warm to medium high-heat, adding coconut oil once it has warmed. Then, add the onions and cook for about 5 minutes, until browned. Add the chorizo and red peppers to the pan, cooking 5-10 minutes. The onions should be translucent and the chorizo should be crisped around the edges.

While you are waiting for the chorizo to cook, add the eggs to a bowl and whisk together with the salt and pepper. Pour the eggs into the pan with the chorizo and cook, stirring occasionally until firm and fluffy. Serve with hot sauce.

Coconut-Cinnamon Pancakes

These delicious pancakes are a little denser than you would expect because it contains only Paleo-friendly ingredients. Still, the flavor is there and they are the perfect substitute when you need to satisfy an early-morning carb craving.

Ingredients (for 4 servings)

- ½ ripe banana (mashed)
- 2 eggs
- 1 ½ tablespoons coconut flour
- 3 tablespoons full-fat coconut milk
- 1-2 tablespoons coconut oil (for frying)
- ½ teaspoon cinnamon
- ½ teaspoon vanilla extract
- ½ teaspoon apple cider vinegar
- ¼ teaspoon baking soda
- 1/8 teaspoon salt

Instructions

Mash the banana in a medium bowl and add the eggs, coconut milk, vanilla extract, and vinegar. Mix until well combined. In a second medium bowl, stir together the dry ingredients. Right before you are ready to cook, add the dry ingredients to the bowl with the banana and eggs and mix until just combined.

Warm the coconut oil in a skillet over medium heat, adding more as needed while you cook. Spoon batter into the pan and cook 1-2 minutes, until bubbles start to form. Then, flip and cook an additional 30 seconds-1 minute on the other side.

Almond Butter and Apple Smoothie

This sweet and tart recipe is so flavorful you don't even taste the spinach. It is rich in vitamins and nutrients, as well as protein.

Ingredients (for 2 servings)

- 2 cups baby spinach
- 1 banana (frozen and chopped)
- 1 Granny Smith apple (cored and roughly chopped)
- 1 cup cold water
- 3 tablespoons almond butter

Instructions

Add all the ingredients to a blender and mix until combined. Continue to blend until the smoothie reaches your desired consistency. You can adjust the amount of water to make it thinner or thicker as well.

Paleo Burger with Eggs and Cashew Cheese

Something difficult to give up on the Paleo diet for some people is most dairy, especially cheese. This cashew cheese makes a substitute in this hearty meal, best served for any meal of the day.

Ingredients (for 4 servings)

- 1 ½ pounds ground beef
- 1 cup raw cashews
- 4 eggs
- Juice of 1 lemon
- 1 clove garlic (minced)
- 4 thick slices tomato
- 4 lettuce leaves (intact)
- Burger seasonings of choice
- ¼ teaspoon salt
- 1/8 teaspoon pepper (or to taste)

Instructions

Start by soaking the cashews 2-4 hours before you are ready to cook. Place them in a bowl and add just enough cold water to cover them. When ready, drain the cashews and put them in a food processor with the garlic, lemon juice, and salt. Blend the cashews until they are smooth.

Then, take the hamburger and create 4 patties. Season with salt, pepper, and any other ingredients you would like. Cook the hamburgers in a large skillet until they reach your desired level of doneness. Remove them from the fan and reserve the drippings. Use the burger fat to cook your eggs until the whites are fully cook (or longer, depending on your preference).

To serve, lay one of the hamburgers on top of a large piece of lettuce. Top each with ¼ of the cashew cheese, a tomato, and the egg. If you want, garnish with minced chives.

Chapter 3: Paleo Main Course Recipes

Smoked Salmon with Dill and Fennel

Salmon and dill is a combination as old as time. These classic flavors come together in this quick and easy dish. It's a great choice if you are just learning to cook salmon because of its simplicity.

Ingredients (for 4 servings)

- 8 ounces smoked salmon (cut into 4 2-ounce pieces)
- 3 large fennel bulbs (diced)
- 4 tablespoons fresh dill (chopped)
- 2 tablespoons coconut oil
- ¼ teaspoon black pepper

Instructions

Heat a skillet to a medium-high temperature. When warmed, add the coconut oil and tilt to distribute. Add the diced fennel to the pan and saute, until tender. This should take about 10 minutes. Then, add the smoke salmon pieces and heat all the way through. Garnish with fresh dill and black pepper before serving.

Garlic-Ginger Pork Tenders over Cauliflower Rice

Spicy garlic and ginger come together in this dish. You should prepare for it ahead of time, allowing at least 2-3 hours (24 is even better) for the marinade to set into your pork. This recipe requires you to cook the rice in some of the remaining marinade, distributing the flavor through the whole dish.

Ingredients (for 4 servings)

- 1 ½ pound pork tenderloin
- 1 cauliflower head (cut into florets)
- 2 tablespoons fresh ginger (2" of the root, sliced)
- 6 green onions (trimmed and sliced)
- 2 cloves garlic (sliced)
- 1 cup coconut aminos
- 1 cup white wine
- 1 tablespoon coconut oil
- 1 teaspoon salt

Instructions

Prepare the pork tenderloin by cutting it into 1-inch rounds. Put it inside a shallow glass dish or a sealable plastic bag. In a bowl, combine the white wine, coconut aminos, and slices of garlic and ginger. Then, pour the mixed marinade into the dish or bag and turn the meat to distribute. When all the meat is covered, seal it and place it inside the fridge for 2 hours to a full day, flipping the meat or squishing it around several times.

Just before you are ready to cook, bring a large skillet to a medium-high temperature. Remove the tenderloin from the marinade, reserving the remaining marinade for later. Use salt to sprinkle both sides of each tenderloin. When the pan reaches temperature, add coconut oil and tilt to distribute. Once the oil smokes, add the tenderloin and cook for 3-4 minutes per side. The internal temperature should reach 145 degrees.

When the meat is cooked, set it to the side and allow it to rest for 5-10 minutes. While you are waiting, make the cauliflower rice. Pulse the rice in a food processor as you normally would. Remove the ginger slices from the marinade and put the marinade in the pan you used to cook the pork. Once boiling, add the 'rice' and cook to heat through, about 2-3 minutes. Serve by placing the rice and sauce on a plate, topped with the tenderloins and sliced green onions.

Paleo Portobello BLT

This recipe substitutes spinach for lettuce and adds avocado to the mix, but you have traditional BLT flavors. The Portobello makes for a hearty, meaty 'bread' for your sandwich.

Ingredients (for 2 servings)

- 4 medium-sized Portobello mushrooms
- 4 slices bacon (cut in half, cooked through)
- 1 cup spinach
- 1 avocado
- 1 tomato (sliced)
- ¼ yellow onion (sliced)
- ¼ cup cashew butter (or Dijon mustard, depending on your preferred taste)
- 1 tablespoon coconut oil

Instructions

Clean the mushrooms and remove the stem. Use the mustard or cashew butter and spread it on the underside of each cap. Then, layer the cooked bacon and vegetables on two of the caps. Top with the remaining caps.

Preheat the broil. Brush the top of the sandwich with coconut oil and place on a tray. Heat 2-3 minutes in the broiler, until toasty.

Danish Meatloaf

This meatloaf uses eggs and almond flour to hold the meat and vegetable mixture together. The tender loaf is contrasted by crispy bacon cooked on top. Serve alongside your favorite vegetable side.

Ingredients (for 4 servings)

- ½ pound ground turkey
- ½ pound ground pork
- 4 bacon slices
- 6 cremini mushrooms (sliced)
- 1 onion (minced)
- 1 egg (beaten)
- ¼ cup full-fat coconut milk
- 1 tablespoon coconut oil
- 1 teaspoon salt
- ½ teaspoon pepper

Instructions

Set the oven to 400 degrees and allow it to preheat while you prepare the meatloaf. Start by adding the coconut oil to a saute pan and warming to a medium heat. Cook the mushrooms and onions for about 10 minutes, until they become tender and start to brown.

While you are waiting for the mushrooms and onions to cook, mix the turkey and pork with the beaten egg, coconut milk, almond flour, and salt and pepper. Allow the mixture on the stove to cool slightly and add it to the meat mixture, thoroughly mixing it in.

Make a large loaf out of the meat mixture and place in an ungreased baking pan. Layer the bacon across the top of the loaf and cook for 50-60 minutes, until the loaf has cooked all the way through and the bacon is crisp. Either discard the drippings or save them for another recipe.

Sweet and Savory Cacao Nip Pork Chops with Butternut Squash

Pork is a versatile meat, making it the perfect pairing to sweetened butternut squash. The cacao nibs add a savory flavor and a slight crunch to the outside of the tender pork chop.

Ingredients (for 4 servings)

- 4 boneless pork chops (about 4-6 ounces each with fat trimmed off)
- 1 medium-sized butternut squash (skin removed, diced)
- 2 cups spinach
- 1 egg
- 1/3 cup raw cacao nibs (chopped)
- 2 teaspoons + 1 teaspoon coconut oil
- 1 tablespoon raw honey
- ¼ teaspoon cinnamon
- 1 teaspoon salt
- ½ teaspoon pepper

Instructions

Use a meat tenderizer to pound on each side of the chops, to make the meat tenderer. In a small bowl, whisk the egg. Dip each pork chop in this, then season with salt, pepper, and the cacao nibs.

Place a saute pan on the stove on medium heat. Add 2 teaspoons of the coconut oil. When hot, add the squash and cook for about 5 minutes, stirring frequently to prevent sticking. Then, place a second pan on a medium-high temperature and warm the remaining coconut oil. Place the pork chops in this, cooking for 3-4 minutes on each side or until they have reached an internal temperature of 165 degrees.

Once you place the pork inside the pan, add the honey and cinnamon to the butternut squash. Cook an additional 5-6 minutes, seasoning with salt and pepper if you would like. Serve the squash on top of a bed of fresh spinach and serve alongside the spinach.

Springtime Pasta with Shrimp and Asparagus

This fresh, summery-pasta is made with Paleo-friendly zucchini noodles (Zoodles) and offers protein from shrimp. It is a great lunch or can be served alongside dinner.

Ingredients (for 2 servings)

- 4 medium-sized zucchini
- 1 pound asparagus (trimmed and cut into 1-inch slices)
- ½ pound shrimp (deveined, peeled, with tails off)
- ¼ pound cremini mushrooms (sliced)
- 2 gloves garlic (sliced)
- ¼ cup white wine
- 3 tablespoons olive oil
- 2 tablespoons fresh tarragon (finely chopped)
- ¼ teaspoon salt
- ¼ teaspoon pepper

Instructions

Start by creating the zucchini noodles. Trim the zucchini. Then, use a mandolin to create julienne 'noodles' or use a vegetable peeler and peel lengthwise. Place the prepared Zoodles in a strainer. Sprinkle with the salt and toss. Allow the noodles to sit at least 20 minutes, tossing periodically. Then, rinse and remove any excess liquid.

Once drained, add olive oil to a large skillet and allow to warm. Then, add the garlic and mushrooms and saute for 3-5 minutes, until the creminis become soft. Put the asparagus in and toss it with the mushrooms and garlic briefly before adding the white wine. Cover the pan and continue cooking for about 2 minutes, until the asparagus starts to become tender and is bright green in color.

Then, add the fresh tarragon, shrimp, and pepper to the pan. Cook an additional 2-3 minutes, until the shrimp is cooked through and bright pink in color. Once the asparagus mixture is finished, toss with the Zoodles and serve.

Beef and Vegetable Asian-Style Wrap

Instead of a highly-processed tortilla shell, this wrap makes use of a crisp piece of Iceberg or Bibb lettuce. Flavors like fish sauce, coconut aminos, ginger, and select vegetables come together for an Asian experience.

Ingredients (for 2 servings)

For the wraps:

- 1 pound ground beef
- 6 large lettuce leaves (intact)
- ¼ head green cabbage (shredded)
- 4 button mushrooms (sliced)
- 2 cloves garlic (minced)
- 1 onion (chopped)
- 1 tablespoon fresh ginger (chopped)
- 1 tablespoon fish sauce
- 1 tablespoon coconut aminos
- 1 tablespoon apple cider vinegar

For the garnish:

- 2 green onions (chopped)
- 1 carrot (shredded)
- ¼ head green cabbage (shredded)

Instructions

Warm a skillet to medium heat and add the onions and ground beef. Cook about 7-8 minutes, until thoroughly browned. Then, stir in the ginger and garlic, cooking for an additional 1-2 minutes until fragrant.

Next, add the cabbage and mushrooms and cook for 5-6 minutes, until they become soft. Stir in the fish sauce, aminos, and vinegar and cook an additional minute, until heated all the way through.

Set this to the side and assemble the garnish by tossing the ingredients together in a bowl. Spoon the beef mixture into lettuce leaves and top with the vegetables for garnish.

Coconut and Lemongrass Chicken Drumsticks

These tender wings have the fresh flavors of coconut water and lemongrass. They are also made in the crock pot, which means less work for you and low risk of your meat overcooking.

Ingredients

- 10 chicken drumsticks (skin-off)
- 4 cloves garlic (minced)
- 1 cup + ¼ cup coconut milk
- 1 stalk (about 5-inches) lemongrass (trimmed, with the outer skin removed)
- ¼ cup green onions (chopped)
- 3 tablespoons coconut aminos
- 2 tablespoons fish sauce
- 2-3 inches fresh ginger
- 1 onion (thinly sliced)
- 1 teaspoon five spice powder
- 1 teaspoon salt
- ½ teaspoon pepper

Instructions

Add the chicken drumsticks to a Ziploc bag or a large bowl and coat with the salt and pepper. Set to the side. Then, add 1 cup of the coconut milk, coconut aminos, ginger, lemongrass, garlic, and five spice powder to a food processor or blender and pulse until smooth.

Pour the prepared marinade into the bowl with the chicken and toss to coat. In the slow cooker, layer the onions across the bottom. Then, add the chicken and marinade on top. Cook on low heat for 4-5 hours. For a creamy sauce, remove the chicken from the crock pot when done cooking and place the remaining marinade and onions in the blender. Add the additional ¼ cup of coconut milk and blend until combined.

Hearty Turkey Chili

Even though chili is thought of as a cool-weather meal, this hearty chili has summer vegetables. This makes it perfect for cool summer nights.

Ingredients (for 4 servings)

- 1 ½ pounds ground turkey
- 4 bacon slices (diced)
- 1 can (28 ounces) crushed tomatoes (no additives)
- 2 medium-sized zucchini (diced)
- 1 onion (diced)
- 1 jalapeno pepper (seeded and minced)
- 2 cloves garlic (minced)
- 1 yellow bell pepper (diced)
- 2 cups chicken stock
- 2 tablespoons parsley (chopped)
- 1 tablespoon chili powder
- 1 teaspoon oregano
- 1 teaspoon cumin
- ¼ teaspoon salt
- ¼ teaspoon chili powder
- 1/8 teaspoon pepper

Instructions

Add the diced bacon to the bottom of a large pot and cook over medium heat until crisp. Remove the pieces with a slotted spoon and place on paper towels to drain. Then, add zucchini, onions, and peppers to the pot with the bacon grease and cook about 7 minutes, until soft. Add the seasonings and minced garlic and cook an additional minute.

Then, stir in salt and pepper and add the ground turkey. Cook about 10 minutes, until the turkey is browned. Stir as it cooks so all the ingredients are mixed together. Once cooked, add the chicken broth and canned tomatoes. Turn down the heat to a simmer and cook for 30-40 minutes until the chili thickens. Top with the parsley and reserved bacon.

Creamy Broccoli and Chicken Casserole

This casserole is made authentic with crispy almonds and bacon instead of a breadcrumb topping. Its creamy texture is not what you'd expect from a Paleo dish since its void of dairy products, but it is incredibly delicious.

Ingredients (for 4 servings)

- 4-6 ounces of boneless, skinless chicken breasts
- 1 cup full-fat coconut milk
- ½ cup chicken stock
- ¾ cauliflower head (thinly sliced)
- ½ broccoli head (thinly sliced)
- ½ pound white button mushrooms (sliced)
- 4 bacon slices (diced and cooked until crispy)
- ½ cup almonds (sliced)
- 1 egg
- 1 tablespoon coconut oil
- ½ teaspoon salt
- ¼ teaspoon pepper

Instructions

Place a saute pan on the stove and warm to a medium-high temperature. Add the oil once it is warmed. While you are waiting, use salt and pepper to season your chicken. Saute for 7-8 minutes before flipping and cooking the other side until cooked all the way through. When cooked, let the chicken cool until you can handle it and cut into 1-inch pieces.

Set the oven to 350 degrees to preheat. Add the ingredients of the casserole in layers- the broccoli, the mushrooms, the cauliflower, and the chicken.

Use a medium bowl to whisk the chicken broth, coconut milk, and egg together. Once combined, pour this mixture onto the layers and cover with aluminum foil. Place in the oven for 30 minutes. Then, remove the cover and add the almonds and bacon. Bake about 5-10 minutes until the casserole is hot and bubbling and the almonds are lightly toasted. Let the dish sit for at least 10 minutes before cutting, so the liquids set.

Crock Pot Kalua Pig

Traditional Kalua pig takes a whole day to cook over an outdoor smoke pit. Since not all of us have the space (or the time) for this method, this Paleo-friendly Kalua pig recipe has been adapted to the crock pot.

Ingredients (for 10 servings)

- 5 pound Boston pork butt roast (can be bone-in or bone-out)
- 3 bacon slices (thick-cut)
- 5 cloves garlic (peeled)
- 1 ½ tablespoons coarse salt

Instructions

Take the bacon and line the slow cooker with it. Then, place the pork butt on a cutting board and remove the skin if you would like. Salt all the sides of the roast and place it inside the slow cooker on top of the bacon. Roast this for 12-16 hours on the low heat setting. Do not worry about adding any liquid- the roast and bacon fat will make their own.

Once the meat easily falls apart, carefully remove it from the mixture. Shred with 2 forks on a plate or cutting board and place in a large bowl. Test the flavor of the meat. If necessary, add some of the reserved liquid until the Kalua pork is juicy and flavorful.

Roasted Tomatoes Stuffed with Sausage

Sweet, juicy tomatoes are filled with seasoned sausage and roasted in the oven. These are a little small, so 1 ½ tomatoes make up a portion. You can also make them heartier by serving alongside cauliflower rice or another delicious Paleo-side.

Ingredients (for 4 servings)

- 1 pound ground pork sausage (seasoned)
- 6 large tomatoes
- 1 onion (chopped)
- 6 white button mushrooms (sliced)
- 3 tablespoons cilantro (for garnish)

Instructions

Set the oven to 350 degrees to preheat. While you are waiting, place a skillet over medium-high heat and add the sausage, mushrooms, and onions. Cook about 8-10 minutes, until completely browned.

While the sausage is cooking, cut the tops off the tomatoes. Use a spoon to remove the seeds and juices and stir them into the skillet. Place the tomatoes with the bottoms down on a greased baking tray.

Once the sausage is browned, drain the moisture and leftover fat from the pan. Then, spoon it into tomato cups and bake for 10-15 minutes. Garnish with the chopped cilantro before serving.

Crunchy Chicken Fingers

This recipe proves that you don't need grain to enjoy crispy, 'breaded' chicken. Almond flour is baked onto tender chicken in this tasty recipe. You can enjoy these crispy tenders on top of a salad, with a Paleo-friendly dip (you can find some ideas in the next section of the book), or by themselves.

Ingredients (for 4 servings)

- 1 pound skinless, boneless chicken breasts
- 3 egg whites (beaten briefly)
- ¾ cup almond flour
- 1 tablespoon olive oil
- ¼ cup arrowroot powder
- 1 teaspoon salt
- 1 teaspoon cumin
- 1 teaspoon paprika
- ½ teaspoon black pepper
- ½ teaspoon cayenne pepper
- ½ teaspoon garlic powder

Instructions

Start by setting the oven to 375 degrees to preheat. Line a baking sheet with foil and place a wire rack on top. Then, prepare the chicken by cutting it into strips that are 1-2 inches wide. Set these to the side.

Get 3 shallow plates or bowls. In the first, put the arrowroot first. In the second, add the egg whites and whisk them slightly. Add the almond flour and spices in the last bowl and mix to combine. Coat the chicken by covering it in the arrowroot powder and then shaking it off. Then, dip it in the egg whites and dredge it on the flour. Place the chicken directly onto the wire rack and repeat for each individual chicken tender.

When all the chicken is coated, bake it for 20-25 minutes. They should be golden brown, crispy, and cooked all the way through.

Sage-Infused Portobello and Beef Burgers

Flavor is the key component of this savory recipe. Serve alongside your favorite side with some of your favorite burger toppings or place on top of a lettuce wrap with lettuce, onions, Paleo mayonnaise (you can find this recipe in the next section of the book) or whatever other Paleo-friendly ingredients you may enjoy.

Instructions (for 2 servings)

- 1 pound 85/15 lean ground beef
- ¼ pound baby Portobello mushrooms
- 2 tablespoons + 2 tablespoons olive oil
- 3 garlic cloves (minced)
- 2 tablespoons fresh sage (minced)
- 1 teaspoon black pepper

Instructions

Set the oven to preheat to 350 degrees as you clean the mushrooms. Then, cut them into quarters and set on a baking sheet. Bake for 15-20 minutes, until the mushrooms cook down to half their size. While you are waiting, add 2 tablespoons of the olive oil to a skillet over medium heat. Add the sage and garlic and cook for 2-3 minutes.

Add the sage and garlic mixture to a food processor. When they are done, add the roasted mushrooms as well. Process until the mushrooms are coarsely chopped. Add this mixture to a large bowl and combine with the hamburger and black pepper until combined.

Warm the skillet you used to fry the garlic and sage to warm the remaining 2 tablespoons of olive oil over medium heat. Cook for about 5 minutes on each side, until cooked all the way through.

Rosemary Grilled Chicken Breast Wrapped with Bacon

The savory flavors of rosemary and garlic are grilled into this chicken breast. It's wrapped with a strip of bacon for added fat. Serve with your favorite Paleo-friendly side.

Ingredients (for 4 servings)

- 1 pound skinless, boneless chicken breasts
- 4 thick bacon slices
- 8 sprigs fresh rosemary
- 4 teaspoons garlic powder
- 1 teaspoon salt
- ½ teaspoon pepper
- Oil for the grill grate

Instructions

Oil the grill grate and set to medium-high heat. Allow it to preheat while you prepare the chicken breasts. Use the garlic, salt, and pepper to season the chicken. Then, place 2 sprigs of rosemary on each breast. Use a slice of bacon to hold the rosemary in place, securing with a toothpick if necessary.

Place the chicken on the grill for 8 minutes before flipping and cooking an additional 8 minutes. Cook until the temperature is 165 degrees internally and there is no pink in the middle.

Creamy Coconut Clam Chowder

This chowder pairs a creamy broth of coconut with protein-rich clams and bacon and filling sweet potatoes. It is hearty enough to be eaten for lunch or dinner.

Ingredients (for 6 servings)

- 1 cup chopped clams (drained, with liquid reserved)
- 2 medium-sized sweet potatoes
- 1 can full-fat coconut milk
- 6 bacon slices
- 2 celery stalks (chopped)
- 2 carrots (sliced)
- ½ onion (diced)
- 2 cloves garlic (minced)
- 2 tablespoons arrowroot powder
- 2 tablespoons olive oil
- 1 tablespoon fresh parsley (chopped)
- ½ teaspoon Italian seasoning
- ½ teaspoon salt
- ½ teaspoon pepper
- ¼ teaspoon cayenne pepper

Instructions

Add the sweet potatoes, celery, and carrots to a large pot and add just enough water to cover them. Cook on medium high heat for about 10 minutes, until tender. Set this to the side, without draining the liquid.

As you are waiting, cook the bacon over medium heat. Remove from the pan and place on top of paper towels or a rack, so the grease drains. Add the onions and garlic to the bacon grease. Cook about 5-7 minutes, until the onions are soft. Then, push this over to one side of the pan and add the clams on the other. Saute for about 4 minutes, being careful not to overcook.

When the clams are cooked, remove them and the onions to the pot with the sweet potatoes and veggies. Then, crumble the bacon into the pot.

Next, use a small pan to heat the arrowroot powder and lard over medium low heat. When well combined, slowly add the coconut milk. Stir the mixture constantly until it thickens, being sure it does not come to a boil. Stir in the seasonings when hot and then add the coconut milk mixture and the clam juice that was reserved to the pot. Heat the pot until the chowder is hot, but be careful that it does not come to a boil or your soup will burn.

Beef and Liver Mediterranean-Style Eggplant

Liver has a distinct taste, making it a food that not everyone enjoys. Still, mixing the liver with beef as you do in this recipe and using Mediterranean flavors allows you to get all the nutrients of liver without the strong taste.

Ingredients (for 4 servings)

- 2 medium-sized eggplants
- ¾ pound ground beef
- ¼ pound veal liver (ground)
- ½ cup walnuts (toasted, chopped)
- 6 tomatoes (diced, with juices retained)
- 1 onion (diced)
- 2 cloves garlic (minced)
- 2 tablespoons fresh mint (chopped)
- 1 tablespoon balsamic vinegar
- 1 teaspoon oregano
- ¼ teaspoon salt
- 1/8 teaspoon pepper

Instructions

Set the oven to 400 degrees to preheat. Cut the eggplants, long ways. Use a sharp knife to score the flesh of the eggplant, being careful not to pierce the skin. Create a crisscross pattern inside the eggplant, with each line about 1" apart from the others going the same direction.

Use the olive oil to coat the flesh of the eggplant. Then, lay with the flesh-side down on a baking sheet and put in the oven for 25-30 minutes, until the eggplant becomes soft and tender.

While you are waiting, add the liver, beef, garlic, and onion to a skillet and brown over medium heat. When cooked all the way through, add the tomatoes and oregano to the mixture. Turn down the temperature to a simmer and stir in the salt and pepper. Cook until the tomatoes start to break down, about 10-15 minutes. Then, stir in the balsamic vinegar.

Once the eggplants are cooked, top with the beef and tomato mixture. Sprinkle the chopped mint and walnuts on top when you are ready to serve.

Cilantro Lime Pork Tacos

Bright flavors come together in this dish. The perfectly seasoned pork and toppings are placed on top of a crisp butter leaf, the perfect substitute for a processed tortilla shell.

Ingredients (for 4 servings)

- 8 large butter leaves (intact)
- 1 pound pork tenderloin (fat trimmed and cut into thin strips, less than 1/2-inch each)
- 2 tomatoes (diced)
- 2 avocados (peeled, pitted, and sliced)
- 1 red onion (diced)
- 1 jalapeno pepper (seeded and minced)
- ½ cup chicken broth
- 3 tablespoons fresh cilantro (chopped)
- 3 tablespoons lime juice
- ½ teaspoon salt
- ¼ teaspoon pepper

Instructions

Use the salt and pepper to season the pork strips, tossing them to coat. Then, warm a skillet to medium-high heat and add the coconut oil. Once it starts to smoke, add the pork and cook 4-5 minutes, until lightly browned. Set this aside in a bowl.

Use the same pan to cook the onion and jalapeno. Be cautious of adding jalapeno seeds to the pan, since they will smoke. If you want jalapeno seeds for added heat, stir them in once the jalapeno and onion mixture is tender, about 5-7 minutes.

When the onion is tender, stir in the broth and tomatoes. Allow this to simmer over a low heat for 2-3 minutes, scraping the bottom of the pan to knock the browned bits loose. Then, add the pork and accumulated juices to the pan. Stir in the lime juice and cook 5-10 minutes, until the pork has cooked all the way through.

To serve, place the pork mixture inside the butter leaves. Add avocado slices and chopped cilantro before serving.

Paleo Supreme Pizza

Sausage, vegetables, and Paleo-friendly crust come together in this tasty recipe that will satisfy your pizza craving. Plus, who doesn't love pizza?

Ingredients (for 2 servings)

- 1 cup almond flour
- 1 sausage (cut into ½ inch thick slices)
- 2 eggs (beaten)
- 4 white button mushrooms (sliced)
- 2 cloves garlic (minced)
- 1 red bell pepper (diced)
- ½ cup grape tomatoes (halved)
- ½ cup no-sugar added marinara sauce
- 3 tablespoons almond butter
- 2 teaspoons + 1 teaspoon olive oil
- ½ teaspoon fennel seed
- ½ teaspoon oregano
- ½ teaspoon salt

Instructions

Set the oven to 350 degrees to preheat. Add the almond flour to a bowl with the beaten eggs, almond butter, and salt. Use 2 teaspoons of the olive oil to grease a baking sheet. Spread the pizza 'dough' until you form a ¼"-inch thick crust. Put this in the oven for 10 minutes.

While the crust is cooking, add the rest of the olive oil to a skillet and bring to medium-high heat. Cook the sliced sausage, mushrooms, and onions until the sausage becomes brown and the onions and mushrooms start to become tender. Set this to the side and use the pan to cook the red pepper and garlic for 3-5 minutes, until just tender. Do not overcook any of the vegetables, since they will cook longer in the oven.

When you are ready to remove the crust from the oven, carefully cover it with the marinara sauce. Add the vegetables and sausage to the top and sprinkle with fennel seed and oregano. Return to the oven for about 20 minutes. Then, add the halved tomatoes to the top of the pizza and bake an additional 5-10 minutes. Use caution when lifting this out of the pan, since the crust will not firm up quite as much as traditional pizza dough.

Chapter 4: Paleo Sides, Soups, Dips, Dressings, and Salads

Zucchini Fritters

These tasty bites make a great snack, or a side to a burger or chicken dish. You can alter the recipe by adding ingredients like bacon, green onions, broccoli, or other veggies. Plain yogurt and homemade guacamole (or mashed avocado) taste great as a dip or a topping.

Ingredients (for 2 servings)

- 3 eggs
- 2 medium-sized zucchini
- 2 tablespoons bacon grease (or coconut oil)
- 1 tablespoon coconut flour
- 1 teaspoon salt
- ¼ teaspoon black pepper

Instructions

Prepare the zucchini by hand-shredding it or roughly chopping it in a food processor, depending on how you want the consistency of your fritters. Set to the side on a plate, blotting with a paper towel if the zucchini is especially wet.

Crack the eggs into a large bowl and whisk together. Then, sift the coconut flour in and mix together. Add the shredded zucchini, salt, and pepper to the bowl and mix to combine.

Set the fritter mix to the side while you warm a cast iron skillet over a medium-low temperature. Add the grease (or oil) once the skillet has warmed. Then, create fritters and fry them in the grease, a few minutes per side until browned and cooked all the way through.

Avocado-Cilantro Dressing/Dip

This recipe makes a great dip or dressing. It is packed full of healthy fats from the avocado and flavor from lime and cilantro.

Ingredients (for 8 servings)

- ¾ packed cup fresh cilantro (chopped)
- 2 green onions (chopped)
- ½ avocado (skinned and pitted)
- 1 clove garlic
- 1/3 cup avocado oil
- ¼ cup lime juice
- ¼ cup full-fat coconut milk
- 1 teaspoon salt
- ½ teaspoon pepper

Instructions

Add all the ingredients to a blender and mix until all the ingredients are smooth and combined. If the consistency is too thick for your preference, add additional olive oil or coconut milk. You can store leftovers for about 4 days, but you will need to blend before serving since the ingredients will separate.

Sautéed Sweet Potatoes

Sweet potatoes are one of the high-carb foods that you can eat without feeling guilty on the Paleolithic Diet. This is a hash-brown style dish that goes great alongside eggs for breakfast or a meat for lunch or dinner.

Ingredients (for 2 servings)
- 1 large sweet potato (grated)
- 1 tablespoon coconut oil
- ¼ teaspoon cinnamon
- 1/8 teaspoon nutmeg

Instructions

Place a skillet on a stove to a medium temperature. Once warm, add the coconut oil. Tilt the pan slightly to disperse and add the grated sweet potatoes. Sprinkle the cinnamon and nutmeg on top and stir to combine. Then, saute on either side until tender, cooking longer if you want them to be browned like traditional hash browns.

Basic Salad Dressing

This recipe provides a base that you can add different herbs to as you learn what you like on different Paleo salads. Some good options include chives, tarragon, rosemary, thyme, basil, oregano, and chives. Since you can easily adjust the recipe for the flavors you want, choose any combination of herbs and create something that tastes great to your palate.

Ingredients (for 8 servings)

- 1 cup extra virgin olive oil
- 1 clove garlic (minced)
- ¼ cup balsamic vinegar
- 1 tablespoon lemon juice
- 1 teaspoon herb or herbs of your choice (adjust as needed)
- 1 teaspoon raw honey
- 1 teaspoon Dijon mustard
- 1 teaspoon salt
- ½ teaspoon pepper

Instructions

Add the balsamic vinegar, minced garlic, lemon juice, honey, and mustard to a medium bowl and mix together until they are all well incorporated. Alternatively, you could use a blender. Once they are mixed, slowly add the olive oil as you continue to whisk or blend.

Next, taste the dressing. Add the salt and pepper, as well as the herbs. Adjust until you reach your desired taste. This dressing can be stored in an airtight container for as long as a week.

Apple Coleslaw

Tangy Granny Smith apples, crisp cabbage, and sweet bell peppers come together in this recipe. This is coated with a sweet and tangy dressing.

Ingredients

- ¼ cup olive oil
- 1 Granny Smith apple (peeled, cored, and grated)
- ½ cabbage head (chopped)
- Juice of 1 lemon
- 1 red bell pepper (chopped)
- 1 celery stalk (chopped)
- 2 tablespoons raw, organic honey
- 1 ½ teaspoons celery seed
- ½ teaspoon salt

Instructions

Add the prepared apples, cabbage, bell pepper, and celery to a large bowl and toss to combine. In a separate bowl, whisk together the remaining ingredients. Pour this over the fruits and vegetables and stir gently to combine.

Creamy Garlic-Pepper Dip

This creamy dip recipe tastes great as a spread for Paleo bread, a dip for veggies or chicken tenders, on sandwiches, and more. You can alter the flavor with different herbs if you choose.

Ingredients (for 4 servings)

- 1 cup raw cashews
- ½ cup olive oil
- 2 cloves garlic
- 2 tablespoon nutritional yeast
- 2 tablespoons lemon juice
- 1 teaspoon pepper
- ½ teaspoon salt

Instructions

Add the cashews to shallow dish. Add cold water until it just covers them and soak for 3-4 hours. Be careful of over-soaking, because this will alter the flavor of the cashews.

Once you are ready, drain the water from the cashews and add them to the blender with the other ingredients. Process until completely smooth. If it seems to thick, you may need to add a little water to the blender. Adjust the seasoning as needed and blend again. Then, store in an airtight container for up to 3 days in the refrigerator.

Shrimp Cakes

Healthy fats and nutrients from assorted vegetables come together in these delicious cakes. They can be served as a side or even an easy meal.

Ingredients (for 4 servings)
- 1 pound shrimp (de-veined, peeled, with tails off)
- ½ cup almond flour
- ½ cup fresh cilantro (chopped)
- 1 egg
- 2 green onions (thinly sliced)
- 1 red bell pepper (diced)
- 2 garlic cloves (minced)
- 3 tablespoons coconut oil
- 1 tablespoon raw honey
- 1 tablespoon lime juice
- ½ teaspoon sea salt
- ¼ teaspoon ground chipotle

Instructions

Process the shrimp in a food processor until it is finely chopped. Add this to a large bowl with the green onions, pepper, egg, honey, lime juice, cilantro, garlic, and chipotle. Mix well and then create patties that are ½-inch thick. If your mixture is not thick enough, you can add a little almond flour to the mixture.

Once the patties are formed, warm a large skillet and add the coconut oil. When it reaches a medium temperature, add the patties and cook for about 5 minutes on each side until brown in color. Place on a plate lined with paper towels and cook the remaining patties.

Paleo Langostino Lobster Squat Soup

This is a spin on a traditional Mexican soup with tender Langostino lobster pieces, vegetables, and a spicy, savory broth. If you cannot find lobster, this recipe tastes equally delicious when made using shrimp. Either way, it contains plenty of protein and healthy fats.

Ingredients (for 4 servings)

- 2 pounds shelled Langostino lobsters
- 2 cans (6.5 ounces each) chopped clams
- 2 cups water
- 1 cup chicken broth
- 1 can (14.5 ounces) crushed tomatoes (no sugar added)
- 2 carrots (peeled and diced)
- 2 garlic cloves
- 1 onion (chopped)
- 2 large-sized mild-flavored dried chilies (like Guajillo or Anaheim chilies)
- 1 bay leaf
- 1 teaspoon dried oregano
- 1 teaspoon olive oil
- 4 teaspoons cilantro (chopped, for garnish)
- 1 lime (quartered, for garnish)
- 1 teaspoon salt
- ½ teaspoon pepper

Instructions

Add the dried chilies to a bowl and add just enough water to cover them. Soak for 30 minutes. Then, remove from the water, remove the stems, and take out the seeds. Add the chilies to a food processor with the canned tomatoes, garlic, onion, and oregano and blend until pureed.

Next, add the olive oil to a pot and warm over medium-low heat. After it has warmed, add the puree and cook at a simmer for 6 minutes, until fragrant. Next, add the juice from the cans of clams, water, chicken broth, and the bay leaf. Continue to simmer for an additional 5 minutes so the flavors can muddle together.

While the soup base is simmering, prepare the carrots and rinse the Langostinos. Add the carrots and simmer an additional 5 minutes. Then, add the clams and lobsters. Once the pan returns to a simmer, cover with a lid, turn off the heat, and let it sit for 10 minutes. This slow-cooking will flavor the sea food without turning it rubbery and overcooking it.

Taste the soup once 10 minutes has lapsed and add the salt and pepper, using the recommended amounts or adjusting as needed. Additionally, you could add hot sauce or dried red chili flakes if you want additional spice. Before serving, top with the chopped cilantro and 1 of the lime wedges.

Creamy Mushroom Soup

You would think any 'cream' of soup would be off limits, since they involve dairy. This recipe uses avocado to make it creamy, as well as to add healthy fats. The mushrooms and other vegetables also give it plenty of vitamins and nutrients.

Ingredients (for 2 servings)

- 6 white button mushrooms (sliced)
- 2 medium avocados (peeled, with pit removed)
- 1 red bell pepper (diced)
- 2 tomatoes (diced)
- ¼ onion (minced)
- 2 cloves garlic
- Juice of ½ medium-sized grapefruit
- 1 cup water
- 1 cup chicken stock
- 4 tablespoons fresh basil
- 1 tablespoon coconut oil

Instructions

Place the water and chicken stock on the stove and bring to a boil. When hot, add to a food processor with the avocado, garlic cloves, and grapefruit juice. Pulse until it is a smooth consistency and set to the side.

Place a medium pot on the stove and warm to medium-high heat. When warmed, add the coconut oil. Then, put the remaining ingredients in the pan and saute until softened, about 8-10 minutes. Add the mixture from the food processor and cook until hot.

Garlic-Ginger Almond Dressing

This dip/dressing pairs well with chicken, seafood, and other meats. It has Asian-inspired flavors and offers the perfect blend of spicy and sweet. You should note that because of the sesame oil, this is best served without heating.

Ingredients (for 6 servings)

- 5 tablespoons coconut aminos
- 1 green onion (minced)
- ¼ cup sesame oil
- 2 tablespoons almond butter
- 2 cloves garlic
- 1 tablespoon raw honey
- 1 tablespoon fresh ginger (minced)

Instructions

Add all the ingredients to the blender until thoroughly mixed. Always blend just before using, since the oil will cause all the ingredients to separate. This tastes great on vegetables, meat, or salad.

Sweet Potato Fries

These sweet, salty, and crisp fries are the perfect pairing for grilled chicken, a hamburger, or even on top of a steak salad.

Ingredients (for 4 servings)

- 4 medium-sized sweet potatoes
- 3 ½ tablespoons olive oil
- ½ teaspoon salt
- ½ teaspoon cumin
- ¼ teaspoon black pepper

Instructions

Set the oven to 400 degrees to preheat. Lay a sheet of parchment paper on a baking tray. Cut the potatoes into fries, with or without skin, about ¼-inch thick.

Add the cut sweet potatoes to a large bowl with the olive oil and seasoning. Toss to coat and place in a single layer on the baking tray. Do not overcrowd, because this will make your fries soggy. Bake for 15 minutes and flip before baking an additional 15 minutes. The sweet potato fries should be lightly browned and crisp.

Roasted Roots Ratatouille

Root vegetables are at the heart of this savory dish, with pine nuts for crunch and a little added protein. This makes a great snack or a side to a meat of your choosing.

Ingredients (for 4 servings)
- 1 eggplant (diced)
- 2 sweet potatoes (peeled and diced)
- ½ butternut squash (peeled and cubed)
- 2 carrots (diced)
- 1 zucchini (diced)
- 1 red onion (chopped)
- ¼ cup toasted pine nuts
- ¼ cup fresh parsley (chopped)
- 2 tablespoons olive oil
- 1 teaspoon fresh thyme
- ¼ teaspoon salt
- 1/8 teaspoon pepper

Instructions

Set the oven to 400 degrees so it can preheat. Then, prepare a baking tray by lining it with a sheet of parchment paper. Add the carrots, butternut squash, and sweet potatoes to the tray and toss with olive oil and the herbs. Then, cook in the oven for 15 minutes.

Carefully add the remaining vegetables to the tray and stir. Return to the oven to roast until the vegetables have browned lightly and become tender. This should take 20-25 minutes. Just before serving, mix the roasted vegetables with the pine nuts.

Italian-Style Garlic and Herb Spaghetti Squash

Plump tomatoes, slices of garlic, and select herbs give an authentic Italian taste to this side. It pairs especially well with a main dish of chicken or shrimp.

Ingredients (for 4 servings)
- 2 pounds spaghetti squash (about 1 medium squash)
- 1 cup grape tomatoes (sliced)
- 2 cloves garlic (thinly sliced)
- 2 tablespoons olive oil
- 1 tablespoon fresh basil (chopped, for garnish)
- 1 teaspoon parsley
- 1 teaspoon salt
- ½ teaspoon black pepper

Instructions

Start by setting the oven to 375 degrees to preheat. While you are waiting, prepare the spaghetti squash by cutting it in half. Use a spoon to remove the seeds and place the squash in a baking dish, with the cut side down. Add water until it is about 1/2 an inch high. Cook in the oven for 35-40 minutes, until the squash becomes tender.

Once the squash is cooked, allow it to cool. When you can handle it, use a fork to scrape the squash flesh out, trying not to squish the strands of squash. Set these on a plate, off to the side.

Then, warm the olive oil to medium heat in a large skillet. Add the garlic and cook for 1-2 minutes, being careful not to brown it. Then, add the halved tomatoes and parsley to the pan and cook another 2 minutes, until the tomatoes are soft and warm. Remove the pan from the heat and add the spaghetti squash, tossing to combine. Top with fresh basil before serving.

Simple Cauliflower Rice

For many people, rice is a difficult staple to give up when they go Paleo. With its flexible flavor and ability to be textured like rice, however, it is not packed full of carbohydrates.

Ingredients (for 4 servings)

- 1 cauliflower head (with most of the stem removed, cut into florets)
- 2 tablespoons coconut oil
- 1 tablespoon salt
- 1 teaspoon pepper
- Seasonings of your choice (depending on the recipe, you could use ginger, garlic, curry, lime juice, cilantro, or any other seasoning)

Instructions

Add the cauliflower florets to a food processor and pulse until it has a coarse consistency, similar to rice. Do not over-process. Season with salt, pepper, and your choice of seasonings and pulse once more to combine.

Then, place a large skillet on the stove and bring it to a medium-high temperature. Add the coconut oil and tilt to distribute. Then, add the cauliflower and saute for 4-5 minutes, until the cauliflower is tender and warmed all the way through.

Paleo Mayonnaise

Mayonnaise is the perfect complement to a sandwich. Unfortunately, it is not usually Paleo friendly. This easy-to-make version always thickens and can be stored for up to a week in the fridge in an airtight container.

Ingredients (for 8 servings)

- 2 large, pastured egg yolks
- ½ cup avocado oil
- ½ cup extra virgin olive oil
- Juice of ½ lemon
- 1 teaspoon Dijon mustard
- ¼ teaspoon salt

Instructions

Add the avocado and olive oils together in a bowl and set to the side. In a separate bowl, add the lemon juice to the egg yolks. Use a hand mixer or quickly beat the ingredients to blend. Slowly add in the oils, continuing to blend a small drizzle. You will need to beat for at least 4-5 minutes for the oil to be completely incorporated. When you have a thick mixture, blend in the mustard and salt until well incorporated.

Paleo Egg Drop Soup

Chinese food is probably one of the biggest no-nos on the Paleo Diet, especially since it usually contains high levels of MSGs and other processed ingredients. This doesn't mean that you can't enjoy it with the right substitutions though and this egg drop soup is proof of that.

Ingredients (for 2 servings)

- 3 cups chicken stock
- 2 eggs
- 2 teaspoons fish sauce
- 1 teaspoon hot chili peppers (thinly sliced, for garnish)
- 2 teaspoons fresh cilantro (chopped, for garnish)
- 2 scallions (thinly sliced, for garnish)
- ½ teaspoon salt

Instructions

Add the stock to a medium sauce pan and warm to a medium-high heat. Add the fish sauce and salt, adjusting as needed. Once it has reached a rolling boil, it is time to add the eggs.

Place the eggs in a small bowl and whisk together until well-combined. If you would like, you can add more salt and fish sauce to the eggs to taste. Once the eggs are ready, remove the soup pot from the heat. Slowly whisk in the eggs- they should cook as they come into contact with the broth, making thin and wispy egg strands rather than chunks. Top with the chili peppers, scallions, and cilantro and enjoy.

French Dressing

This sweet and savory dressing is the perfect complement to a salad, which is great since most retail dips are not approved for the Paleo Diet.

Ingredients (for 6 servings)

- 1 can (6 ounces) tomato paste (minimally processed)
- 3 tablespoons Paleo mayonnaise (recipe can be found on the previous page)
- ½ cup olive oil
- ¼ cup raw honey
- ¼ cup champagne vinegar
- ¼ onion (chopped)
- 1 clove garlic
- 1 teaspoon paprika
- 1 teaspoon Worcestershire sauce
- ¼ teaspoon salt
- ¼ teaspoon pepper

Instructions

Add all the ingredients except the olive oil to a blender. Process until it has a smooth consistency. Then, slowly add the olive oil and blend an additional 2-3 minutes, until completely incorporated. This stores for as long as week.

Paleo Bread

This recipe has a hearty, grainy flavor like most breads, but it is grain-free and Paleo-friendly. You can enjoy it toasted for breakfast or use it to make a tasty sandwich.

Ingredients (for 10 servings)
- 3 cups almond flour
- 7 eggs
- 6 tablespoons flax seeds (ground)
- 3 tablespoons coconut flour
- 1 ½ tablespoons raw honey
- 1 ½ tablespoons coconut oil (melted, plus more for coating the pan)
- 1 ½ tablespoons apple cider vinegar
- 1 ½ teaspoons baking soda
- ½ teaspoon salt

Instructions

Start by setting the oven to 350 degrees to preheat. Use a stand mixer (or a food processor) to combine the ground flax, two types of flour, baking soda, and salt. Pulse until well combined. Then, mix in the eggs and mix until combined. Finally, add in the remaining ingredients.

When well mixed, prepare a bread pan by greasing it with coconut oil. Use a spatula to help you scrape all the batter into the pan. Bake for 30-40 minutes, until the bread is cooked all the way through and you can insert a knife into the center and have it come out clean. If the top browns too much, you can put a sheet of foil over it while it finishes cooking. Let the bread cool completely before slicing it.

Broccoli Soup

This nutrient- and vitamin-packed soup has rich broccoli flavor that is enhanced with chicken broth, lemon, and bacon. Even without the cheese that is usually found in this type of soup, it is hot, creamy, and delicious.

Ingredients (for 4 servings)

- 3 broccoli heads
- 5 cups chicken stock
- 2 small turnips (quartered)
- Juice of 1 medium lemon
- ¾ cup unsweetened almond milk
- 1/3 cup full-fat coconut cream
- 8 bacon slices (cooked and crumbled)
- 1 onion (chopped)
- 2 tablespoons coconut oil
- ¼ teaspoon salt
- 1/8 teaspoon pepper

Instructions

Place a large soup pan on the stove and warm the chicken stock. As its warming, heat a skillet to medium heat and melt the coconut oil. Add the turnips, onions, lemon juice, and salt and pepper to the skillet and cook for 5 minutes, until the vegetables are slightly softened.

Then, stir the broccoli into the skillet and continue cooking for 5 minutes. Turn down the heat to a simmer and stir in the chicken broth. Cover this and simmer for 10-15 minutes, until the broccoli becomes tender. Then, add the heated mixture to a blender and process until it has a smooth consistency. Mix in the almond milk and coconut cream before returning to the stove, in the pot you used to heat the chicken stock. Heat over medium-low until hot all the way through and top with bacon crumbles.

Chapter 5:
Paleo Snacks and Desserts

Bacon Wrapped Dates

This recipe is baked, bringing out the sweet dates to contrast beautifully with the crispy, salty bacon. Four of these bites makes a filling snack! To keep the bites from unraveling while they cook, pierce them with toothpicks before putting them in the oven.

Ingredients (for 4 servings)

- 16 Medjool dates
- 8 slices bacon (halved)
- 16 whole almonds

Instructions

Set the oven to 375 degrees to preheat. Then, use a knife to slightly open a date. Press an almond inside each. Then, wrap half a strip of bacon around the date. As you wrap these, place on a baking tray with the seam of the bacon facing down. Cook for 7 minutes. Then, flip and cook an additional 7-10 minutes, until the bacon becomes crispy. These bites taste great warm or cold.

Coconut Cashew Cream and Banana Tart

The sweet, tropical flavors of this dish come together on top of a Paleo-friendly crust. Delicious cashew cream and coconut fill this pie and bananas are assembled on top.

Ingredients (for 10 servings)

- 1 ½ cups dates (pitted)
- 1 ½ cups pecans
- 1 cup cashews (soaked and drained)
- 4 bananas (firm, but ripe)
- ¾ cup unsweetened coconut (shredded)
- ½ cup water
- 1 vanilla bean (split open and scraped)
- 2 tablespoons + 2 teaspoons maple syrup (plus more to taste, if needed)

Instructions

Add the pecans and the salt to a food processor and pulse until coarsely chopped. Then, add the dates and pulse about 15-20 seconds, just until well combined. Finally, add the syrup to the blender and pulse until combined. The mixture should stick to itself slightly. This will be the crust of the pie- press it into a 9-inch pie plate and set to the side.

Next, make the filling. Grind the cashews in the blender until they have a coarse consistency. Add the vanilla scrapings, water, and syrup to the cashew mixture and blend until smooth. You want the filling to have a consistency similar to very thick pancake batter. Remove 2 tablespoons of coconut for the garnish and put the remainder in the blender, mixing until just combined. Use this to create an even layer in the prepared piecrust.

Slice the bananas, using a slightly diagonal angle. Use the banana 'coins' to create round rows, starting at the crust and slightly overlapping as you move inward. Top with the remaining coconut and serve.

Guacamole Deviled Eggs

Rich avocado and cooked egg yolks in this spin on a traditional deviled egg. This meal is packed full of healthy fats from the avocados and protein from the eggs for a filling snack or side.

Ingredients (for 2 servings)

- 1 large avocado
- 4 eggs (hard-boiled)
- 1 teaspoon lemon juice
- ½ teaspoon hot pepper sauce (or to taste)
- 1 ½ teaspoons red pepper flakes (or to taste)
- 1/2 teaspoon salt
- ¼ teaspoon black pepper

Instructions

Slice the avocado in half and pit it, before removing the flesh to a food processor. Slice the eggs the long way, removing the yolk and adding it to the food processor with the avocado.

Set the egg whites to the side and add the hot sauce, pepper flakes, lemon juice, salt, and pepper to the processor. Then, pulse the ingredients until combined and your desired consistency. You can puree until smooth or leave chunky. Use a spoon to fill the egg whites with the guacamole mixture and enjoy.

Spiced Pumpkin Seeds

This recipe offers traditional fall flavors with something that is always around in the fall- pumpkins! This is a great snack to munch on regardless of where you are. The ingredients for this list are non-specific, since you can use the basic recipe to create small or large batches. You can also change the spices and herbs used to change the flavor.

Ingredients (for 10 servings)

- Raw pumpkin seeds from 1 pumpkin
- 1 tablespoon allspice
- 1 tablespoon cumin
- 1 tablespoon coriander
- 2 tablespoons olive oil
- ½ teaspoon salt
- ½ teaspoon pepper

Instructions

Set the oven to 350 degrees to preheat. Boil water in a large or medium pot, depending on the size of your batch, with 1-2 teaspoons of salt to the water. Take the innards of a gutted pumpkin and remove the seeds, cleaning off the bits of pumpkin as you go. Place them inside a strainer and rinse using cold water, until there are no stringy bits or pumpkin meat left on them. They should be white in color.

Once the water has reached a boil, add the seeds and cook for 10 minutes. Strain them through the strainer and rinse. Then, pat the seeds dry using a towel. Add the dried seeds to a large bowl and add 1-2 teaspoons of olive oil. You want them evenly coated, but just barely. Add the spices and toss all the ingredients together.

You may need to do more than one batch of pumpkin seeds, depending on how many you are making. Lay the seeds in a single layer on a baking tray, overlapping them as little as possible. Roast in the oven for 10 minutes and stir. Then, bake the seeds 5-10 minutes longer, carefully removing a few of the seeds and cracking them open to be sure the insides aren't burning (they will be brown if they are). You will know the seeds are done when the outsides are lightly browned and easy to bite through.

Dehydrated Apple Chips

These apple snacks have a crunch. After being slow cooked in the oven, they are dried out. Cinnamon and fresh-squeezed apple juice give this recipe flavor, but you can easily make them with another juice or with other seasonings.

Ingredients (for 4 servings)

- Juice of 5-6 large apples (about 2 cups)
- 2 large apples
- 1 cinnamon stick
- 1 teaspoon cinnamon

Instructions

Set the oven to 250 degrees to preheat. Add the apple juice and cinnamon stick to a large pot and allow it to come to a low boil. Core the 2 apples and remove the tops and bottoms. Cut into slices that are about 1/8-inch thick.

Then, drop the slices into the boiling juice. Cook until the apple slices look translucent, about 4-5 minutes. Take a slotted spoon and carefully remove the slices from the juice. Place on a cloth towel and gently pat dry.

Then, place the chips on a wire cooling rack over a baking tray. The tray will catch excess drips. Bake 30-40 minutes in the oven, until the apples are almost dry when touched and golden brown in color.

Chocolate-Coconut No-Bakes

These no-bake cookies will remind you of a Mounds bar, but without the processed ingredients. You can make the cookies as large or as small as you like, just remember that ¼ of the recipe is a serving.

Ingredients (for 4 servings)

- 1 cup unsweetened coconut flakes
- ½ cup dark chocolate chips (at least 85% dark)
- ¼ cup almond butter
- ¼ cup unsweetened cocoa powder
- 3 tablespoons coconut oil
- 2 tablespoons raw honey

Instructions

Add the chocolate chips and coconut oil to a microwave safe bowl and cook 30 seconds at a time, stirring after each interval until thoroughly melted. Then, stir in the honey, almond butter, and cocoa powder until smooth. Once smooth, stir in the coconut flakes.

Set the mixture to the side while you prepare a baking sheet by covering it with parchment paper. Drop the prepared mixture onto the sheet, using a tablespoon or ice cream scoop. Refrigerate the cookies until they harden.

Cucumber Salmon Bites with Cashew Cheese

Crisp cucumber, smoked salmon, and creamy cashew cheese come together in this recipe. These delicious bites are a great snack, especially since they are best eaten cold.

Ingredients (for 4 servings)

For the bites:

- 1 pound smoked salmon
- 1 medium cucumber
- 2 tablespoons fresh chives
- Cashew cheese

For the cashew cheese:

- 1 ½ cups raw cashews
- ¼ cup water
- Juice of 1 lemon
- 1 clove garlic
- ¼ teaspoon salt

Instructions

Make the cashew cheese first. Set the cashews in a bowl and cover them with the water, using more if needed. Let them sit for 3-4 hours. Then, drain them and put the cashews in a food processor.

Add the remaining ingredients for the cashew cheese to the blender and process until it has a smooth and creamy texture. You can add a little water if needed to thin the cheese, depending on your desired consistency.

Slice the cucumber into 1/4-inch thick rounds. Add some of the cashew cheese and a tablespoon of salmon to each bite. Place these on a tray and sprinkle with the chives when you are finished.

Easy Watermelon Freeze

This sweet and cool treat is perfect for a summer day. The addition of mint makes this recipe even fresher and provides the watermelon with a contrasting flavor.

Ingredients (for 2 servings)

- 4 cups unseeded watermelon (cubed)
- 1 cup water
- Juice of 1 lemon
- ½ medium cantaloupe (cubed)
- 3 tablespoons fresh mint

Instructions

Add the cantaloupe and watermelon to a food processor and blend until smooth. Then, put the mixture into a saucepan over medium heat until it simmers for about 15 minutes.

When the watermelon mixture is almost done, place the mint into another saucepan and cover with the water. Bring to a boil and steep for 3 minutes. Then, strain out the mint leaves and add the water to the melon mixture. Remove the mixture from heat and stir in the lemon juice.

The mixture is now ready to freeze. You can use paper cups, an ice cube tray, or popsicle molds. If you are using a cup or a tray, let the mixture firm up for about an hour before inserting the popsicle stick. Freeze completely, about 4 hours before serving.

Sweet Potato Brownies and Chocolate Icing

This is definitely not a dessert you'd expect to be eating on the Paleo Diet. It is rich in chocolatey flavor. While the sweet potatoes give the brownies their moist texture, you cannot taste them at all in this recipe.

Ingredients (for 12 servings)

For the brownie:

- 1 large sweet potato (baked and peeled)
- 1 cup unsweetened cocoa powder
- 2 tablespoons coconut flour
- 2 eggs
- ½ cup coconut oil (melted)
- ½ cup raw honey
- 1 tablespoon baking powder
- 1 tablespoon vanilla extract
- ½ teaspoon baking soda

For the icing:

- 1 cup dark chocolate chips
- 1/3 cup coconut oil
- 1 tablespoon vanilla extract

Instructions

Set the oven to 365 degrees to preheat. Mash the sweet potatoes and add them to a large bowl with the coconut oil, eggs, honey, and vanilla. Mix to combine. In a separate bowl, add the coconut flour, cocoa powder, baking soda, and baking powder and combine. Stir the dry ingredients into the bowl with the sweet potato mixture.

Set the bowl to the side while you lay parchment paper inside an 8x8 pan. Spread the batter evenly across the bottom and place in the oven for 25-30 minutes. It is done once a toothpick can be inserted and comes out clean. Do not overbake or your brownies will not be as moist.

Once you put the brownies in the oven, start preparing the frosting. Add the coconut oil and chocolate chips together in a pan on the stove. Mix together over low heat until melted and then stir in the vanilla. Remove the pan from the stove and transfer the frosting to the refrigerator. It will need to cool completely before the next step.

Take the frosting and use a hand mixer to whip it until it becomes fluffy. When the brownies are done, allow them to cool before topping with the icing and servings.

Paleo Trail Mix

Trail mix is a great snack, since it requires no preparation, does not need to be refrigerated, and can be enjoyed anywhere. You can use this recipe or alter it slightly to meet your own taste preferences.

Ingredients (for 12 servings)

- 2 cups raw pumpkin seeds (unsalted)
- 2 cups sunflower seed kernels (roasted, unsalted)
- 1 cup almond slivers (roasted, unsalted)
- ¾ cup dried coconut flakes (toasted)
- ¾ cup dried pineapple (diced)

Instructions

Add all the ingredients to a large bowl and toss to combine. Store in an airtight container and enjoy!

'Ice Cream' Bites

These chocolate-covered 'ice cream' bites are sure to satisfy your cravings. The best part about it is they are Paleo-friendly so you don't have to feel guilty about eating a few.

Ingredients (for 6 servings)

- 3 medium-sized bananas (cut into 1-inch pieces and frozen beforehand)
- 7 ounces 80% or higher dark chocolate (finely chopped)
- ¼ cup coconut oil
- 3 tablespoons almonds (toasted and chopped)
- 1 teaspoon vanilla extract
- 1/8 teaspoon salt

Instructions

Add the frozen banana pieces and vanilla extract to a food processor and combine until the mixture is smooth and creamy. Then, place the ice cream in a sealed, airtight container and freeze for 2-3 hours, until it solidifies.

Use a teaspoon or small ice cream scoop to make the balls. You want to have about 24 to eat 4 of the ice cream bites for a serving. Line a baking tray with parchment paper and place the balls on this. Once you are out of ice cream mixture, return to the freezer so they don't melt while you prepare the chocolate.

Add the coconut oil and chocolate shavings and cook in a double boiler until melted. Alternatively, you could microwave for 20-30 seconds at a time until smooth. Use a skewer or fork to pick up each ball and dip it into the chocolate mixture. Top with a few toasted almond pieces and return to the tray. Allow to set for 10-15 minutes in the freezer (or until solid) before eating.

Bacon-Tomato Sweet Potato Bites

Crispy and salty bacon comes together with juicy tomatoes and soft sweet potato for a medley of flavors. They taste good warm or cold, so make some ahead and keep them in the refrigerator for whenever you are hungry.

Ingredients (for 6 servings)
- 2 medium-sized sweet potatoes
- 2 cups grape tomatoes (quartered)
- 6 bacon slices (chopped and crisped in a skillet)
- ¼ cup fresh parsley (chopped)
- 2 tablespoons olive oil
- ¼ teaspoon salt
- 1/8 teaspoon pepper

Instructions

Warm the broiler to the high heat setting and lay a piece of parchment paper on a baking sheet. Slice the sweet potatoes into slices that are 1/8-inch thick. Use half the olive oil to coat the top of the sweet potatoes and sprinkle with the salt. Put these in the broiler until they are slightly charred on top and softened.

While you are waiting, add the remaining olive oil to the crisped bacon, tomatoes, and parsley and toss. Spoon this on the sweet potato slices and season with pepper before serving.

Strawberry Rhubarb Crisp

This sweet and tangy dessert resembles all the flavor of a strawberry-rhubarb pie, but it is free of processed sugar. Instead, natural honey and date sugar are used as sweeteners and the crumble is a gluten-free version.

Ingredients (for 4 servings)

- 2 cups fresh strawberries (cleaned and sliced)
- ½ pound rhubarb (peeled and diced)
- ¾ cup almonds (finely diced or coarsely ground)
- ¾ cup coconut oil
- ½ cup unsweetened applesauce
- ½ cup coconut sugar
- ½ cup starch or tapioca flour
- ¼ cup raw honey
- ¼ cup date sugar
- 1/8 cup coconut flour

Instructions

Set the oven to 400 degrees so it can preheat. Add the strawberries and rhubarb to a large bowl with the raw honey, date sugar, and almond flour. Stir to combine. Use oil to coat a 9x9 baking dish and spread the prepared mixture inside. Set this to the side.

Use a medium mixing bowl to combine the 2 flours with coconut sugar, diced almonds, coconut sugar, applesauce, and coconut oil. Stir all the ingredients are distributed throughout. Bake for 35-40 minutes, until the strawberries and rhubarbs have softened and the top has started to brown.

If you choose, you can top with coconut whipped cream. (You can find this recipe next). You can also garnish with fresh slices of rhubarb or strawberries.

Coconut Whipped Cream

Since traditional whipped cream is full of dairy and sugar, you would assume it's something you have to give up on the Paleo Diet. As you choose your coconut milk, be sure it is full-fat. You want to be able to separate the fatty oils of the coconut from the liquid.

Ingredients (for 4 servings)

- 1 can full-fat coconut milk (chilled in the fridge overnight, upside down)
- 1/8 teaspoon cinnamon or nutmeg (optional)
- 1/8 teaspoon vanilla extract (optional)

Instructions

If you turned the can upside down to refrigerate the coconut milk, then it should be separated with the oils on top. Remove the oils and reserve the remaining liquid for another recipe or discard. Add the solidified oil to a medium bowl and use a wire whisk or electric beater to beat it until it starts to form soft peaks. Add in the vanilla and cinnamon if you are using them and continue to beat until the coconut cream reaches your desired consistency.

Almond Macaroons

This delicious, buttery recipe melts in your mouth. It offers plenty of almond taste and satisfaction for your sweet tooth with a Paleo-friendly recipe.

Ingredients (for 6 servings)

- 1 ¼ cups almonds
- 2 egg whites (beaten)
- ¼ cup raw honey
- 1 teaspoon lemon juice
- 1 teaspoon lemon zest
- 1/8 teaspoon cinnamon

Instructions

Set the oven to 250 degrees to preheat. Use a food processor to coarsely chop the almonds, being careful not to over-process and make a paste. Set these to the side.

Add the lemon zest and cinnamon to a medium bowl and mix. Add the beaten egg whites to this mixture and then stir in the lemon juice and honey. Beat until the ingredients are fully incorporated. Then, put the almond mixture in the bowl and blend well.

Take a piece of parchment paper and lay it on a baking sheet. Use a teaspoon to create mounds of the almond mixture. When you run out of dough, bake for 30 minutes. For easy removal, use a spatula to take the macaroons off the paper while they are slightly warm.

Chia Seed Pudding with Coconut and Pecans

This sweet recipe is easy to throw together and even so filling that you could eat it for breakfast. You can eat it about 2 hours after preparing but you should refrigerate overnight if you want the chia seeds especially soft.

Ingredients (for 4 servings)

- 2/3 cup chia seeds
- 3 cups full-fat coconut milk
- 1/3 cup unsweetened coconut (shredded)
- 1/3 cup pecans (chopped)
- 1 teaspoon raw honey
- 1 teaspoon vanilla extract

Instructions

Add the chia seeds to an airtight container or a mason jar and mix with the coconut milk, honey, and vanilla. When stirred well, seal and place in the refrigerator for at least 2 hours. Just before serving, stir in the coconut and pecans. Top with a few extra pieces of each to garnish.

Conclusion

Thank you again for downloading this book!

I hope this book was able to help you to realize some of your health goals using the Paleolithic Diet. Whether you are looking to lose weight or just to improve your overall health, the recipes and guidelines provided in this book can help you.

The next step is to clean the junk food out of your house and replace it with some of the nutrient-rich, wholesome foods to make the Paleo Diet recipes in the book. You have the knowledge, now the rest is up to you!

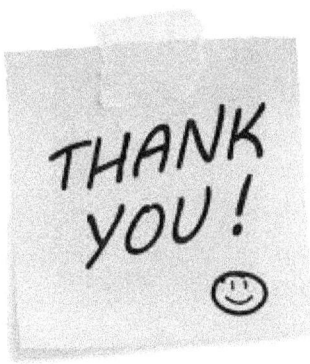

Finally, if you enjoyed this book, then I'd like to ask you for a favor, would you be kind enough to leave a review for this book on Amazon? It'd be greatly appreciated!

Thank you and good luck!

Check Out My Other Books

Below you'll find some of my other popular books that are popular on Amazon and Kindle as well. Simply click on the links below to check them out. Alternatively, you can visit my author page on Amazon to see other work done by me.

http://amzn.to/2puTfLc

CrossFit: Barbell and Dumbbell Exercises for Body Strength

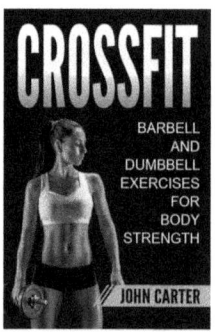

Mediterranean Diet: Step By Step Guide And Proven Recipes For Smart Eating And Weight Loss

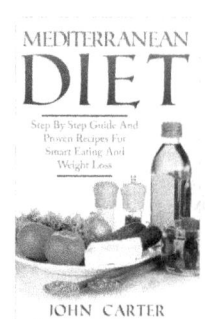

Weight Watchers: Smart Points Cookbook - Step By Step Guide And Proven Recipes For Effective Weight Loss

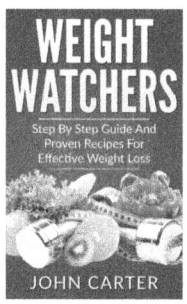

Bodybuilding: Beginners Handbook - Proven Step By Step Guide To Get The Body You Always Dreamed About

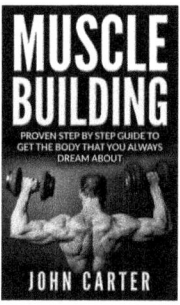

South Beach Diet: Lose Weight and Get Healthy the South Beach Way

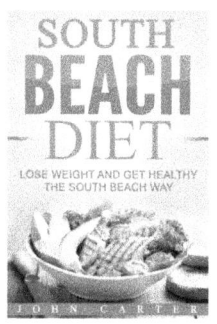

Blood Pressure: Step By Step Guide And Proven Recipes To Lower Your Blood Pressure Without Any Medication

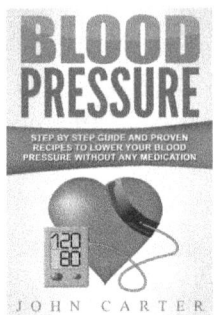

Meal Prep: 65+ Meal Prep Recipes Cookbook – Step By Step Meal Prepping Guide For Rapid Weight Loss

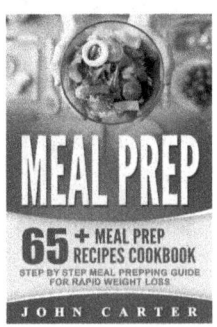

If the links do not work, for whatever reason, you can simply search for these titles on the Amazon website to find them.

www.ingramcontent.com/pod-product-compliance
Lightning Source LLC
Chambersburg PA
CBHW070031040426
42333CB00040B/1534